T0209530

Other Books:

Mercy, Lord, Mercy

Spirit of a Sound Mind

A Broken-hearted Schizophrenic

CAT Meows 2

Changes Deranges

goin', goin', gone

In the Mood for Food

A Mess in Distress

Catherine E. Goin

WESTBOW
PRESS®
A DIVISION OF THOMAS NELSON
& ZONDERVAN

WestBow Press books may be ordered through booksellers or by contacting:

WestBow Press
A Division of Thomas Nelson & Zondervan
1663 Liberty Drive
Bloomington, IN 47403
www.westbowpress.com
844-714-3454

Interior Image Credit: Catherine E. Goin

Scripture taken from the New King James Version®. Copyright © 1982 by Thomas Nelson. Used by permission. All rights reserved.

ISBN: 978-1-6642-6106-8 (sc)
ISBN: 978-1-6642-6105-1 (hc)
ISBN: 978-1-6642-6104-4 (e)

Library of Congress Control Number: 2022905093

Print information available on the last page.

WestBow Press rev. date: 04/25/2022

Dedicated :

Russell Goin without whom I could not publish my books
Deborah Heckman who helped me with my book
Dr. David Goldstein in charge of my mind/ body
Cindy Rafala, a counselor who helps me with relationship
Randy Michener, my art teacher for many years

Quote from Oscar Wilde from "The Picture of Dorian Gray"

"It is only shallow people who don't judge by appearances. The true mystery of the world is the visible, not the invisible."

Genesis 3: 21 NKJV the David Jeremiah Study Bible

"Also for Adam and his wife the Lord God made tunics of skins and clothed them."

Contents

Chapter 1

A Mess in Distress

I confess that under duress
I was a mess in distress,
Which Dr. Lebensohn found appalling and galling.
What I should do was unknown to me—
A complete mystery.
I didn't look good—or feel good, for that matter.
My appearance and my brain
Were all a-scatter—sort of like the Mad Hatter.

This book is about the importance of appearance—whether man, woman, or child. I learned this lesson the hard way and will never forget it so long as I live and have some control over my mind.

Way back when I began life on this planet wandering around the cosmos, the USA had only two months earlier entered the infamous conflict known as World War II, which followed closely behind World War I and the Great Depression. Almost everything was rationed, and people for the most part were sorely lacking in money and goods. Beauty parlors and clothing stores were limited, and their products were not easily available. I grew up with my grandmother and mother making my clothes, taking into consideration that material was not readily available. When I was a young girl, Mom, Granny, and I would go into Washington, DC, and look at the windows of Hechts, Kanns, and Garfinkles to see what was in fashion. Granny was a talented seamstress and would then go home, cut out a pattern, and make what she had seen. The thrift shop was where the wealthier members of our community would take their slightly worn clothing. Lerners, Graysons, Carters, the BonTon, and the Fashion Shop were the only clothing stores on Main Street, if my memory serves me correctly.

Cars were not commonplace. My uncle Lawrence and my father shared a car for a long time. Russell and I walked to school, which was fun and something youngsters today do not usually get to do. We were left to our own devices and consequently grew up with a highly developed sense of adventure. Pants were not common for girls and women. Mostly, we wore dresses and skirts with blouses and sweaters. Tennis shoes were available, as were loafers with leather soles that always needed to be replaced. And for girls, there were Capezio ballet flats, which I loved. Jeans were not worn everywhere as they are today.

My mother whacked off my hair as the hair salons in the area were out of our price range. When COVID hit, and things closed once again, I started snipping off my hair. It doesn't look any worse.

We were expected to look appropriately attired when attending school. Nobody (poor, middle class, or rich) could look slovenly. Getting dressed was fun and an event I loved doing every morning. That is undoubtedly when I first became interested in fashion and style, grooming, and the importance of how one looked. Our posture was so important that as young girls and women we would walk around our rooms with a book on our head, which rarely fell to the floor. I recently started doing this again, but the books fall to the floor.

Clothes were relatively modest, and instead of being skintight, skirts were intended to slide easily over the hips. As I got older, I started wearing pants—not jeans but slacks. When I graduated from college, jeans started appearing everywhere.

Chapter 2

Old Age and Style

It's another day, and the clock says 2:30 a.m. ...and I go walking off into the early morning air. My mind's sole concern is what to wear for the day.

I think the new Patagonia gray pants with the facial expressions of Darth Vader will do. The pants are a little long, a look I like but one not compatible with my advanced age and instability. They're about an inch too long, which might cause me to stumble and fall. That's how I damaged the bone in my right hip, which then had to be totally replaced. Bummer! Now it takes concentration to exercise— walk, yoga, weights, aerobic machines, and so forth. I must learn to walk properly to get through the day without falling. The weights are largely to gain muscle, which then helps protect my bones.

Back to style. The Patagonia pants and Darth Vader T-shirt came from Hope Heals, where I volunteer, which I love because I am surrounded by clothes of all sorts for all genders, ages, and sizes. It's like being in heaven. I find some of the coolest stuff there. I give them money since they provide clothing for people who otherwise may not have it.

Why do I love clothes so much? Probably because I painted and drew for fifty years and love visual beauty, texture, line, and color. These elements excite my spirit. My grandmother and mother were enthusiastic about clothes also, causing me to start out my life loving clothes and fashion. My first memory of style was a pair of red jeans, which at the time were quite avant-garde as most females did not wear pants. I was around six or eight. The war was over, and articles of apparel were becoming available once again. I loved those jeans!

The Darth Vader T-shirt is fun. Someone had a goofy sense of humor. It is a boy's shirt but fits, so I wear it with joy. I wear it and the Patagonia pants with my black Croc ballet flats, which are about the only dressy shoes I can wear that don't hurt my feet. My days of three-inch spikes are long gone, a remnant of the past. This outfit goes perfectly with my Native American silver bear earrings that I got at Déjà Vu, the coolest consignment shop in town.

In addition to being fun, caring for your appearance is important because that is a factor in how people make and form their impression of you—usually in their first seven to thirty seconds of seeing you. This impression is difficult to change. I know I judge people that way and should know better, but I do attempt to find the good in people and compliment them. If they make the effort a compliment should be forthcoming.

Hopefully my appearance isn't boring. That would be too gross and depressing for words.

Chapter 3

Style! Style! Style!

It takes a while to develop, to envelop one's heart,
To start to love one's apparel so as not to quarrel,
Which injures the expression of one's face?
Adding to the disgrace of an injured being—
One not capable of seeing
What there is in front of one's eyes—not so wise!

So begins my approach to the art of fashion, especially developing an individual style, which we should protect and allow to flourish to the best of our ability. Hopefully, we will find a mentor, a guru. Preferable more than one. Guides!

How do you find these gurus?

1. Look around you. Look at the people you admire for their gracefulness and generosity of spirit. Their unique approach to fashion is a manifestation of their hearts.

2. Look at magazines, the media, *General Hospital,* and the movies. The media is somewhat limited as they are rarely fashion-forward, which to my mind is an essential part of one's approach to style and fashion. One of my favorite mentors has been Stacey London. She and Clinton Kelly hosted *What Not to Wear,* one of my favorite TV shows that I watched for ages. It enchanted and instructed me. They took into consideration all types of problems that men and women encounter. In my present case, that no longer is excess poundage but being short (should I say petite?) and old is. A young saleslady said to me as I pondered buying a piece of attire that seemed too youthful for me, "Betsy, fashion has no age." She was being a good salesperson but probably honestly believed what she said. I bought the article.

3. As for a modern guru, I admire Peggy Cappy, whose realm of expertise is yoga, which is important for good style in my opinion. Her DVDs and TV shows help me to maintain good posture, which is difficult for someone almost eighty. Yoga, walking, exercise, and even meditation help me to maintain good posture and an erect spine. These areas inspire me to make my best effort.

4. To be kind, tell those who look nice that they do. A sincere compliment can make a person's heart soar and spirit roar. We live in such an antagonistic, stress-driven world that hearing something nice is wonderful and brings a smile to the face. It certainly does for me, and I never forget to say, "Thank you," to the person who encourages me.

5. Knowing you look nice is good for your being. Cavemen and cavewomen wanted to look appealing, not to mention warm. God, in His wisdom, adorned them with animal skins when they were kicked out of the Garden of Eden, lo those many eons in the past. Today we don't need to use animal skins as there are many wonderful

fabrics used to make clothing stylish and warm. Animals need their skins. We don't need their skins. God created these animals because He loves them as well as us. They add beauty and diversity to the world, characteristics we need.

Chapter 4

Fashion Is Infinitely Interesting

Fashion to me is infinitely interesting. It seems that men control the fashion industry. Women, though, seem to understand what women want and need better. They are not so cutting-edge, but when it comes to parting with one's hard-earned cash for a piece of apparel and then wearing it more than one time, I tend to go for what women design. I ask myself after each wearing "Do I love this piece of clothing enough to wear it another time?" If not, I recycle it. I no longer can drive distances to malls and other shopping areas, so I need to shop locally which in my case involves two regular shopping stores and what is available is consignment and thrift shops. I manage to look cutting edge by doing this.

Resources are limited and there are billions of people in the world competing for them. Therefore, it behooves us to care for our resources and when we can, reuse and recycle them. If we are tired of our clothes or they no longer fit our figures or lifestyles, see to it that someone else can get them and love them and use them. This goes for my other love, books! If I am not going to read them again or even for the first time, then I donate them someplace where others can get them and enjoy them rather than taking them to the dump.

Now, and for the last several years distressed items have been all the rage. My brother says that when men wear their clothes to rags and throw them in the trash designing women recover them and sell them for a small fortune. He says that sometimes he's embarrassed to be seen with me. One must be careful though. The holes and distressing needs to be in the absolute perfect location or they won't be any fun. When old skin showing through is not appropriate, the problem is solved by patches. I take everything to Yumi, my favorite seamstress, who is outrageously expensive but does such a lovely job it's worth every penny. Since I don't have a sewing machine or a place to sew Yumi solves the problem of alterations for me. She is Asian and there is possibly some Zen in her. After all these years of meditating, reading, painting it seems that there is a Zen streak in me ... a little bit of Zen, a little bit of Zat keeps one from getting fat ... she knows I love clothes and likes to work with me, so I give her free reign.

Back to recycling: It seems to be the hottest rage for the last ten years or so all over the world. I know when we get tired of things in the USA, we should send them to areas deprived of garments. In my travels it is apparent that women in most countries have an eye for color, design, texture and line and manage to pull off 'looks' from clothing we no longer want to wear ... "What goes around comes around."

As for jewelry the expensive stuff usually bores me silly. I like funky, unusual items. Today I bought the coolest necklace for a mere $5. I find diamonds boring even though they sparkle which should appeal to the crow in me, but they don't.

As for shoes ... about all I can wear in my advanced years are my black, Croc ballet flats. They don't hurt my feet and they fit, for which I am thankful and delighted to wear them. They are rubber and last forever. Every now and then I discover something else in the way of footwear that is comfortable and that I can walk in.

Why must women suffer by wearing or trying to wear clothes men tend to design for the tall and very thin and rich among us. Their motto should be, "No lives matter, only money matters."

Onward with style ... to make the world smile ... go away cursed ones who espouse ugliness and lack the ability to admire the loveliness of God's creation.

A Black Skirt

As I recall I had one black skirt which was A-line and just past the knee cap. I wore it everywhere. My favorite skirt though was a blue plaid kilt which I wore with my royal blue Capezio ballet flats. I paid for them by sitting with kids whose parents were gone for the evening. This started when I was around 13 and continued until I was old enough to work at Grayson's for more money and more shoes and skirts. Looking back, I don't remember jeans.

Jeans didn't become part of life until the 60's. Thank you hippies! Until you appeared on the scene there were basically no jeans. Denim was mostly for farmers and was found most often in overalls. And then ... lo and behold ... bell bottoms which were a gift to the flower children and hippies and me. Today they don't seem so cool because jeggings and skin-tight leggings are favored. They are okay but too tight on my calves for me to be comfortable and happy. My legs prefer loose pant legs as does my entire psyche. This probably goes back to the words immortalized by the designer of my first uniform. His name escapes my mind, but his words have guided me throughout my entire adult life. "What did he say?" you may ask. Well, as he was adjusting the length of my skirt he looked up and deeply into my eyes and said …"Miss Goin, tight clothes are not quite nice!" He would be horrified by what he would see today. Almost everybody wears their clothes so tight that every roll of fat is visible and wobbles when people walk. Ease of movement obviously means nothing to them, but after years of dance, walking, yoga, tai chi, and kayaking, etc., it is of supreme importance to me that my body can move with ease and dare I say? gracefully?

To make matters worse many of the jeans are so low cut they slide down over the hips and people are continually hiking them up. One can hardly keep them on and once again rolls of fat hang over them at the waist or what would be a waist if there weren't so many rolls of fat. Even many teens today display this alarming display of fat. It seems that excessive eating is more important than attractiveness and good health. Not to mention the stress caused to the joints—like hips, knees and ankles. I wrote a whole book on food which no longer obsesses me. God made the human body to be useful and beautiful to the eye. It is the temple of the Holy Spirit and to be cared for throughout life. He helped us create clothing to keep warm, modest and attractive. Yet we don't seem to care. How sad!

60 years later everyone is wearing jeans. My favorite is Re-Washed which often is made partially of recycled plastic. I love the feel, and they have a knack for putting the distressed holes in just the right places. Practicality was the original reason for jeans but now the heavy fabric is no longer always necessary. The current trend to more pliable, light weight fabric is much appreciated by me and many others. I love to feel the fabric in my hands and on my body, and

consequently don't enjoy shopping on the computer. If it is pleasing to the touch, to the eye and to the soul—I buy! Today jeans are beloved by almost all of us around the world ... men, women, boys and girls regardless of age and size.

Vive le jeans! Vive le denim! And don't forget denim jackets! And don't forget denim skirts!

Instant Results

Ah, the mystery of life. It begins before birth and extends after death. The mystery of life is not perfect but what is? But what does ones' looks have to do with it.

As Dr. Lebensohn told me, "Miss Goin, you are judged by others in the first 7-30 seconds they see you. This judgement is largely based on your appearance. Their eyes scan you from head to toe, front to back and side to side. What they think is largely based on your appearance. If you look like a slob then to them, you are a slob. And to compound the problem you are scanning them. If you are both slobs, there is no real problem. Overcoming this initial impression is nearly impossible to do."

"That gets back to your impression and your looks in particular." Currently I was starving to death and my hair was a mess … stringy, unkempt and multi-colored because of the lack of a good dye job. I had been trying to grow my hair long which for me is impossible. It was merely stringy and ugly. My eyes were dead! Where had the twinkle gone? Would it ever come back? Schizophrenia is a devastating brain dis-ease and had affected my eyes. Dr. Lebensohn told me he suffered from heart disease which limited his ability to play tennis, which he dearly loved. He told me schizophrenia was no more limiting than his heart disease. But he did tell me I shouldn't starve myself to death as that is a horrible way to go.

So, eat I must! So, eat I did! Dr. Wang and Dr. Lebensohn both encouraged me to eat. It seemed I didn't want to die which was a complete mystery to me. Ah, the mystery of life! It wants to continue. It doesn't want to die. Dr. Wang had turned me into a Follower of the Way of Jesus Christ … a child of God. As a believer I had been promised eternal life in the presence of God, with Jesus as my friend, guide, protector and savior. I had a reason to fight to live!

After my 45 minutes with Dr. Lebensohn, full of agonizing traumas which left me stressed and anxious, he would look at his watch and say, "Miss Goin, this has been interesting but our time is up and you must go. I will see you again soon." He would rise from his chair, extend his hand to help me rise and we would walk outdoors. He would say, "Miss Goin, do stop by Toast and Strawberries (the boutique next to his office) and talk with Rosemary. She will help you with clothing and how to help your appearance." That is precisely what I did!

I walked next door, entered the shop and said "Hi, Rosemary." She was slightly taller than me, pretty, gracious, black and had a beautiful Afro. We would talk while I had fun looking at her. Her shop was exotic, and I loved it and her. She lifted my spirits. When I left, I had a spring in my step, a song in my heart and a shopping bag over my arm.

Style is Free

"Style is Free," ... so says the t-shirt I bought today, along with what I thought were red jeans like I had as a kid. In the sunlight though they were hot pink. I love them and bought a soft orange t-shirt with pink flamingos on the front to go with them. Rosemary would be proud. She was a great mentor all those years I went to see Dr. Lebensohn and Dr. Goldstein, until she either retired or quit. I forget. One day she was gone to be replaced by an upscale tea shop ... not nearly so exciting.

I learned from Rosemary once again the importance of an inquisitive spirit and a good eye. A lot of times when I stopped by to visit, she would have her designer friends in the shop for conferences. They were always polite to me, a honky, and shared their design ideas and tips. I learned to appreciate 'distressed but not a mess.' Cutting the hem and then washing the clothes followed by tumble drying was fun and gave neat end results. I wished to learn to do 'holes' but found that process to be too much complicated work for me ... tedious also.

Her associates had the most revolutionary approach to style to me who had been surrounded most of my life by 'preppies' and 'yuppies' … undoubtedly the most boring dressers in the history of the world. In all fairness I did acquire a love of pink and green and an appreciation of ballet slippers. From Audrey Hepburn came my love of the "little black dress." I also love Geiger jackets.

Meanwhile, I was going to Europe on my trips, spending oodles of time in London, Scotland, Milan, Frankfurt, Paris and Brussels. While most of my inflight buddies were eating pasta, drinking and partying, I was going to concerts, art galleries, design shops and walking for hours on end. In Paris and Brussels, I had the pleasure of hanging out with the sales ladies in the courtier shops. They found in me a kindred spirit with a profound love of beautiful clothes and no money to speak of. We would spend lots of time drinking tea or champagne while watching the runway shows on in-house TV. On occasion I would run into an actual fashion show which was exciting. My favorite one was in Frankfurt. It was outdoors in early fall and the runway must have been a quarter mile long. The models pranced up and down while I drooled in admiration over the gorgeous clothes they wore, especially the dresses which were more beloved by me than my beloved jeans.

One day I stopped into Dior and the sales lady said in her beautifully accented English, "Ah, mademoiselle, there is nothing new since last you were here." She told me about a new consignment shop tucked away on one of the streets nearby where I could get affordable clothing. She, herself, loved to shop there. So off I went to spend my hard -earned dollars.

My special time was on one of my CRAF trips when the crew spent 13 days in Brussels. What a vacation! What an adventure! I discovered a wonderful music store where I stocked up on music for my flute which I had to quit playing after 25 years because of my neck and right side. Now I am learning to play the guitar, the mandolin and the Native American flute.

Thank You for My Freedom

The sensation of movement is essential to well-being. If you were to ask someone incapable of moving freely, like being in a wheelchair, their response would probably affect you profoundly. One's ability to move freely ... dancing, walking, running, biking, etc ... being able to use the body's ability to move with spontaneity is instrumental in the ability to relax.

It is difficult to walk in the morning, enjoy the birds, the breezes, the sun dawning over the land or if walking in the dark to enjoy the stars and the full moon ... like tonight when the Blue Moon is in the night sky. The moon is a never- ending source of pleasure. It is fun to see the deer eating bushes and flowers or to see a fox or coyote running down the street, to hear the birds singing to welcome the coming of day, and the coming of the sun which warms our skin. This is freedom... and the ability to freely walk and talk with your Savior is a joy impossible to surpass. He walked and lived life as should we. Stress destroys this pleasure.

Good shoes are of the utmost importance. If they don't hurt the feet and/or cause blisters they are a source of joy, doing their part in providing this freedom of movement. After my hip injury, total hip replacement and fractured spine I had to learn to walk again, an achievement of sheer determination and pig-headedness. I went to sessions of physical therapy with Blue Ridge Orthopedic and sessions with Nick at OTAC to learn how to work my body at home and at the gym. It was apparent to the physical therapists that I was out of balance, graceless and walking flat-footed. I had to relearn to walk 'heel-ball of foot-toe' and stop looking down and to direct my gaze forward. I could cast my eyes to the ground to avoid stumbling and falling. My neck would go backwards which caused my spine to straighten and my shoulders to fall and come together. I could then walk faster, with more confidence. I am now down to a mile in 28 minutes instead of 38 minutes. That is not as fast as in the past when I was undamaged and younger when I did a mile in 17 minutes … but a definite improvement.

Walking in dresses is fun because they offer the most freedom of movement, being of only one piece of clothing falling from the shoulders. They are comfortable, good looking and easy to move in. When it's cold you can wear tights with the dress and a warm coat or jacket. In winter I look like a Polar Bear but am warm, comfortable and able to enjoy the brisk weather. If it's frigid I cover my face and head with a hat and a mask over my nose and mouth.

One thing that is important is (as my doctor told me) to wear sunglasses to protect the eyes from the rays of the sun. This helps prevent cataracts. One must not look directly at the sun. When I was sick, I walked miles at night into the early morning. I enjoyed the stars and Milky Way which is no longer visible because of light pollution. The last time I saw the Milky Way was when I was at Kitt Peak Observatory. As Dr. Wang said when I landed in the emergency room of the St. Francis Hospital, "Miss Goin, what seems to be the problem?" I said, "The Milky Way turned upside down!" He said, "Things will be okay in the morning!" I passed out.

No Negative Self Talk

"No negative self-talk! We need to avoid it as it leads to anxiety, depression and anger. You have enough of that as it is. That is one of the reasons you ended up in the hospital, in addition to being diagnosed with schizophrenia." So said my doctors ... all of them. How to avoid it? It's difficult to retrain the mind which for years has been taught to hate itself/yourself. You are in the habit of telling your mind and your body they are ugly, worthless, not very bright, etc. and now you think that is true. What to do?

1 ... when angry with yourself think of how it must hurt God to know that you don't appreciate the gift of life He has given you. How must He feel to know that you're not thankful for all you have? For instance, today when going to my mandolin lesson with Mark I met Terry. Terry was in a wheelchair with one leg amputated. While talking to him I discovered that he used to play the guitar and now couldn't because his fingers shook so badly he couldn't use them to play. He also can't hold the guitar. "Betsy, you are so blessed to be able to still walk and as Mark said, "You don't have palsey."

2 ... While talking to Mark, he told me his sister is helping him to lose weight. Mark is smart, extremely musically talented, a funny, intelligent man who happens to be around a hundred or so pounds too heavy. I will pray they are successful and succeed in losing the excess weight.

3 ... I ran into Helen, Patsy's (my cousin) daughter. Helen told me that Patsy is now in a nursing home, totally blind and unable to read Braille anymore. It saddens me to know that I still sometimes feel sorry for myself when I don't have problems like these. I can still read and walk and see and play the mandolin.

These three examples lead me to talk about Dr. Lebensohn's advice to me when I started therapy with him. He said "Miss Goin, every day of your life you are able to get about, go out and talk with people. You will discover you like most people. Most of them have problems and half of them have problems worse than yours." I was floored. He also explained to me that mental illness/brain dis-ease was not shameful, just a disease of the brain instead of the physical body. He suffered from heart disease which caused limitations for him, especially as he couldn't play tennis anymore which he loved. What an eye-opener to me.

So, negative self-talk ... go away! Instead, consider blessings: 1 ... Dr. Wang turned me into a follower of the Way of Jesus. I owe him my soul 2 ... I am creative as are we all and we can see, hear and love beauty, nature and the goodness of others. 3 ... I enjoyed painting for almost 50 years. Now I write and play music. They're different ways of expression but just as meaningful. 4 ... I have a good church.

Remember: as the old song goes, "Count your blessings instead of sheep and you will fall asleep counting your blessings."

Blessed Creativity

Why are we all so self-critical? It is the complete antithesis of being stylish. It is virtually impossible to see only your bad qualities and be fun to look at. I was reading a book about yoga and the author said to stand in front of a full -length mirror (preferably naked if you can stand it) and look at yourself. I invented my words to say: I am blessed, I am big-hearted, and I am beautiful. Repeat this for several minutes. Hopefully these words will sink into your brain and heart, and you will see the beginnings of a great human being who is stylish. After I tried it several times, I began to see what God had created and although I wish He had created me to be tall and thin, I understand He likes variety, and I am what He felt like creating at the time. I am old, tattered and tired, but I am telling my body and brain they have always been good to me; allowing me to walk, talk, do yoga and exercise and given me grace. And I repaid you by saying you were ugly. Finally, I can see my body and brain in all their goodness and to thank them.

As for my brain which is even more complicated… it is horrible to me that I have schizophrenia but after almost 50 years of psychotherapy I have come to peace with my brain and have learned that it, too, has been good to me. It gave me the creativity to paint lovely paintings since around 1960 when I began to study art at the College of William and Mary. To this day my doctors have encouraged me in the pursuit of creativity in all its manifestations. It was fun studying with Drs. Newman, Thorne and Roseburg. Then I studied with Randy Michener at the Manassas campus of NOVA. He was fun and had the wonderful capability to understand his students encouraging them to paint in their own style to the best of their ability. My style was based largely on what I learned from them all:

1 ... if you can draw it, you can paint it.

2 ... don't muddy the colors

3 ... form follows function

"Don't muddy the colors" was especially important when developing a sense of style. Almost any color can be interesting and beautiful if kept clean. Since I love color, this tenet was important to me and my ideas about beauty. It was probably the most important when applied to the development of my style. When I moved in with Russell, I no longer had my studio and there was no room to paint. Giving up painting was not bothersome as I no longer had any thing I wanted to express on canvas. I started to express myself through writing and music (the flute, the guitar and the mandolin). I studied the flute for almost 25 years before I had to quit. After falling twice and damaging my hip and fracturing my spine and hurting my neck I could no longer comfortably hold my flute. I will always love James Galway and Jean Pierre Rampal! The guitar is still somewhat difficult for me to hold but since I got a parlor guitar it is again possible to play it. I like the mandolin the best.

Writing is my greatest love and I wish I had more talent in this area of endeavor. So far, I have self-published 7 books and have 4 more lined up. Then I can die in peace. I am constantly bugged about marketing which I can't afford so I am content with the love of writing and seeing the books in print and in the Library of Congress. I don't have the time, interest or money for marketing.

There are many forms of creativity, as many as there are people. These are talents given to us by God, the ultimate Creator. The body is the temple of the Holy Spirit and should be adorned with as much attention and love it can be given which is a great way to say "Thank You, God

What Rosemary Saw

Over the 30 or so years I visited with Rosemary I learned a lot from her. Not only was she a good businesswoman but she had great style sense. Her friends were leaders of the pack when it came to style and presentation of the self. Rosemary also had the "gift of gab" and used it to fully express herself. At that time, I used painting because talking was difficult for me. I avoided it whenever possible. When around people, though, I followed Dr. Lebensohn's advice. I got out every day and played. Was talking fun? Not really, but it was necessary. I did find people interesting for the most part and creative in a multitude of ways, not just limited to the fine arts and music. Granny used the sewing machine and needles and thread. Mom was a great seamstress as was Granny. They taught me to sew when I was small, and I sewed into my 30's. In Hawaii my apartment was too small for sewing and I had to rely on the stores. When I get to Heaven the clothes will be lovely and I will be in pig-heaven. The people wearing them will also be lovely and interesting. Am I interesting? That's hard for me to know as my former friends, radically conservative, have dropped me and I am making new friends. Hopefully they find me interesting.

So! Back to creativity! I must write! I must write! I must write! Keeping my goal in sight!

What is my goal?

1 ... to do everything I do during the day and night dressed appropriately for the occasion.

2 ... to declutter which helps eliminate stress. This includes decluttering your closets. If you don't love and wear something, give it to someone who will appreciate it. Clothes, shoes and trees need to be loved. They are as 'real' as you and me, and unless annihilated will undoubtedly last as long as we do. Perhaps that is why vintage and consignment shops and thrift stores are so prevalent around the world, appealing to most fashionistas. Buying this way is not so expensive and wasteful of our precious resources. I find beautiful, fashionable and useful clothes which I could never afford otherwise.

Thank You God for seeing to it that I am so well dressed. Please let someone love my giveaways as much as I have loved theirs.

Declutter, You Must

Marie Kondo has made a fortune and become famous telling people to get rid of 'stuff' and not to buy a lot more. I bought two of her books, read them twice and then passed them on. Wayne Dyer said when he moved to Hawaii, he got rid of everything he owned including around 20,000 books and all his attire, sentimental stuff and even photographs. WOW! What a woman! What a man!

Getting rid of a lot of stuff is relatively easy for me. Now when I buy something I have to get rid of something. However, there are about 50 books in my room I don't even let out of my room because I have learned that often they are never returned, and these books are priceless to me. My favorite book in the whole world next to the Bible (KJV and NKJV)is Mikhail Bulgakov's "The Master and Margarita." I have read it about 10 times and think I will read it again as I have not read it for around 10 years.

Now I must address the issue of decluttering one's closets ... including all attire, shoes, accessories, makeup, etc., even though almost everything I wear is recycled. When I get an article of apparel my mantra is "Do I love it enough to wear it again?" If not, I send it on to someone who needs it and will love it. My two closets are small, and it is distressing to see them stuffed. My soul thrives on clean, lean, spare space. I get rid of stuff with regularity, not just seasonally. Since my possessions are now limited to articles I can't easily part with, my shopping has been curtailed. However, as Dr. Lebensohn said, "It's fun and okay to look. It keeps your mind and outlook fresh and stimulated. Never forget Rosemary!" Since my 40 odd years of going to his office at 2015 R. ST., N.W. are over, and Rosemary is gone, I now have Sandra at Déjà vu in Warrenton. She has the coolest consignment shop and the most glorious sense of style, peculiar to European women (she is German). She is savvy about clothing and appearance and has entertained me for over 10 years.

I also admire Lindsey and Tammie who run Hope Heals Free Store where I volunteer. They provide donated clothing and baby items for those who can't afford clothing. There are so many!

It is appalling to me to see all the storage buildings along the road when I go for long drives with Russell. They are everywhere. People buy stuff they have no room for, so they pack it into storage units and then buy more. There are also hoarders. ... my mother was one. They never part with anything and continuously buy more and more and more. It seems there is a deep hole in their heart which can never be filled. They seem to think that possessing a multitude of things will fill this hole, not realizing that 'stuff' can never fill this psychic hole.

I bought a neat pair of blue denim jeggings yesterday for $1. They're wonderful but I can't afford to gain a single pound. Fortunately, I don't have a 'muffin top and can breathe in them. They will be worn with my NASA t-shirt that says, "Is anybody out here?" I also bought a shirt that says, "Life is too short to wear boring clothes."

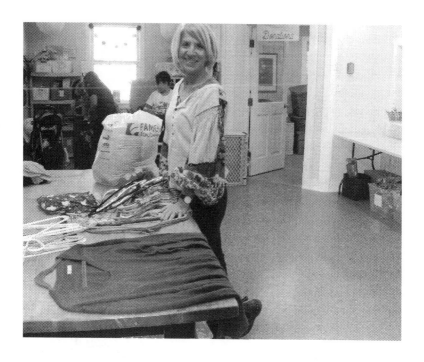

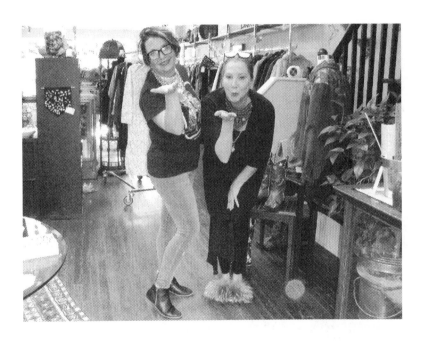

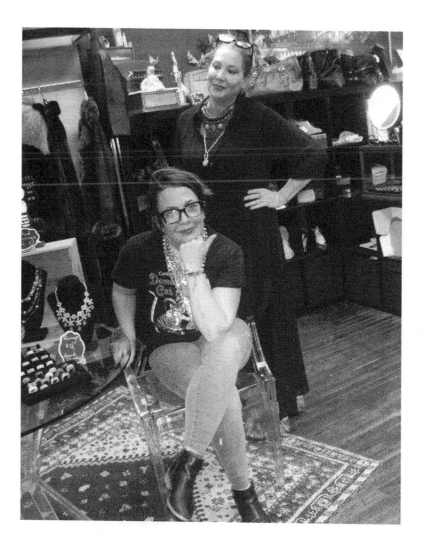

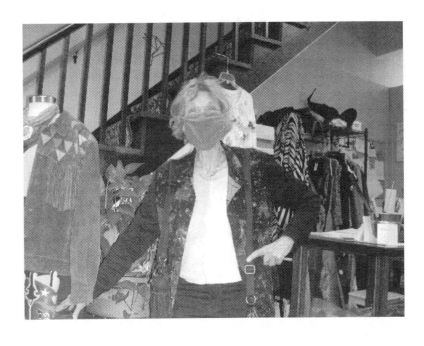

"When you don't Dress Like everyone else... You don't have to think like everyone else."

— Iris Apfel

Style is ageless.

"What Do YOU Want to Do?"

My appearance was under control. After 3 months of eating, I had gained around 20 pounds which satisfied all four of the doctors who had to approve me to go back to work. I had learned to drive and bought a car and was still alive. I had learned most of my approach to driving from what I learned in Paris, which was not to hit the car in front of or beside you, observe the speed limit and park in approved spaces. Rosemary and I had gotten my fashion and appearance in order. I looked presentable.

My hair was acceptable and was a bright red which seemed to suit my sense of self. It was chopped off into a pixie cut which seemed to suit my personality at the time.

The meditation and yoga and walking/exercise seemed to be quieting my mind and talking to people every day helped me cope. Granny had taken it upon herself to help me develop my fashion sense so the two of us would spend time together at her home in Falls Church. We would go to Tysons Corners to go shopping and looking at the latest in what was being worn, especially in the category of my beloved dresses and jeans. Once again, I was in Nordstroms, my favorite store of all time, even more important to me than the shops in Europe.

After our shopping excursion we would go home, sit in front of the TV with a glass of iced tea and watch General Hospital which I loved as much as Star Trek and Star Wars. I learned a lot about how to present myself and how to relate to other people ... so I thought! I loved Bobby and Luke! They both had a highly developed sense of adventure which was of the utmost importance to me at that time. Then we would listen to her favorite music, the Statler Brothers. I wasn't sold on them, but they were okay and the two of us had fun listening together.

The four doctors approved my progress and told me I could go back to work, under observation and staying with my mother for at least six months. That was okay with me as my mother needed my money and I needed a quiet place to rest and recuperate. Besides ... Taffy was there. He was a wonderful white cocker spaniel who was good to me and worthy of every ounce of love he was given. We would talk and walk together along with Wahu. He and Wahu were great friends. Remember Wahu? He was my imaginary dog friend from Hawaii.

Dr. Lebensohn was happy and decided to go to the next step with me. One sunny afternoon he looked me straight in the eyes and said, "Miss Goin, what do YOU want to do?" I looked at him! "What do you mean?" I asked. "I thought you were supposed to tell me what to do!" He said "Think about it ... what do YOU want to do ... not what you think you are supposed to want or what others tell you that you want. Will you think it over?

"I guess so since you put it so nicely!"

How to Picture 'Reality.'

We are finite beings having an infinite experience. This body-mind has infinite possibilities. Deepak Chopra, if I understand him correctlywanys us to:

1 ... understand yourself

2 ... master 'reality'

3 ... go beyond existence

How can that be? Let me see! My story is unique to me, and your story is unique to you ... as unique as we are physically, mentally and spiritually. Although he may not realize it Dr. Goldstein is a master of the mind-body connection. When he took over my counseling around 1998, he seemed to me to specialize in helping me care for this connection. I could finally talk about my past which I only rarely did with Dr. Lebensohn. One day I said to Dr. Lebensohn, "Why don't you have me lie on the couch and do psychoanalysis?" As the old cliché goes "Curiosity killed the cat, satisfaction brought it back."

"Miss Goin," he said, "you don't need to poke around in the past. You are having enough trouble dealing with your present."

Is that what is meant by 'reality?' Being in the present? 'Mindfulness?' It gets a bit confusing thinking about mindfulness and meditation. I seem to live in the present now and have a lot of trouble remembering the past. I feel the pain in my head writing these words about 'reality.' My morning walk and reading of the Bible and morning coffee are my 'reality.' They give structure to my life and provide quiet to my mind. My biggest struggle is what to wear for the coming day.

Today it is my White House/Black Market black capris with embroidered flowers at the hem and my tie-dye t-shirt. I love t-shirts, especially if they tell a story or have a cool picture on them.

Right now, on TV there is CALM's add saying "do nothing for 15 seconds" which I love to do. I hear the falling of the rain ... falling, falling, falling. Is it "going beyond existence?" Did I transcend? I seem to have become 'enlightened' doing Transcendental Meditation. I have spent nearly 50 years doing psychotherapy, being a Christian, and meditating in order to understand myself and my association with my surroundings.

After 16 years the cicadas have reappeared. I hear them in the evening and have seen three dead ones. Is that 'reality?" I also saw a crow swooping into a tree ..."caw, caw, caw!"

That is my reality.

Shop Therapy

I thought and thought about what to do, unsuccessfully for the longest time. Meanwhile Dr. Lebensohn continued his discussion about appearance and one of his favorite topics with me ... Shop Therapy. He said one day, "Miss Goin, you do not need 'shock therapy'. it would probably harm you, but I recommend 'shop therapy,' which is simply the art of looking at and enjoying the beautiful effects caused to your mind by the visual arts ... paintings, fashion, tools, etc. ... wrought by the hands of your fellow brothers and sisters. People are born by the grace of the Creator and each one has been gifted a portion of creativity. It is our job to figure out our type and learn to use it. You have been gifted right now with the visual arts. That is why I suggest you spend time after being with me, at Rosemary's shop, Toast and Strawberries. She is supremely unique and has a wonderful eye for beautiful clothing and jewelry. She has both the gift of displaying them and she has the 'gift of gab.'

Not only is she helping others but is providing an income for herself and her family. Rosemary is a successful human being ... one who is good for you to know. I would like her to be one of your mentors.

One of your other loves seems to be reading and books, so I suggest stopping at Kramer Bookstore on your way to my office. It has all sorts of wonderful books including ones about yoga, meditation and the Creator. As you know, both Dr. Wang and I, want you to meditate. You are way too confused in your mind to reach 'enlightenment' at this stage of your life, but if you are diligent and persevere in learning to understand your 'being' and persevere in our therapy I believe you can achieve enlightenment which will undoubtedly take many years. Your past was destructive, and you need not delve into it now, but you do need to live in the moment. For the present pursue beauty, understanding, and the knowledge of God … His desire for you to love your neighbors as well as loving yourself. You need help with them all."

So back to Shop Therapy: After this visit I stopped by to see Rosemary and enjoyed the time spent with her. She was light-hearted which at the time was all I knew about her.

Light Hearted

I know nothing much about people and their ambitions, desires and attempts to gain self-respect and standing in the community, not to mention the pursuit of material and physical pleasures. What I do know is the result of nearly 50 years of psychotherapy, the pursuit of beauty and the understanding of my faith.

Would I die for it? Yes, in a flash, right this minute. If my unique and unusual contribution to God is to only help one person through my art it would be worth everything I have experienced, encountered and usually lost. But I persevere, probably because I am pig-headed or bull-headed to the nth degree ... something my doctors realized about me.

Has it been worth it? Yes, because now I can laugh, smile, grin, be mirthful and light-hearted like Rosemary ... within. Within what, you ask? I answer in a flash, "why, my shell! My swell shell! That has saved my eternal soul from eternal misery ... read psalm 55: 15-16 NKJV, "Let death seize them; Let them go alive down into hell, for wickedness is in their dwellings and among them. As for me I will call upon God and the Lord shall save me!" If that thought isn't enough to make one light-hearted nothing will.

And that leads us back to appearance. The care, thought and preparation put into presenting yourself before God and your neighbor shows them that you respect and love them. Is that shallow? I think not. If people don't care about presenting themselves in a favorable way, they show no real love for themselves or for other people surrounding them. Even more important than your apparel is your willingness and confidence to smile. After the loss of my smile, it took years of therapy to bring back the twinkle in my eyes. That makes me so happy. And it should you.

You can go in for Shop Therapy, not shock therapy. You can look but not charge. Cold, hard cash if you must buy. That's the way it's meant to be, if it is to be that "style is free", as a t-shirt I saw said. I am going to paint that comment on my new gray t-shirt.

That's all I have to say today. It is now time to meditate on and ponder clothes and fashion … style.

Muffin Top

Muffin tops are one of many can'ts … can't have rolls of fat dropping over the top of one's pants
It's unattractive to behold, especially when one is old
And not comfortable as one has to continuously pull up one's pants which is done unconsciously
A bit unnerving for others to see!

What a topic! It depresses me … the mere thought ought to scare the most cynical among us to tears. Deb had a lot to say about muffin tops last week. So yesterday at 2:30am I hopped out of bed, visions of roles of fat hanging over my jeans running through my head. I was horrified!

De-Clutter … my first thought was "get rid of all of the jeans which are so low cut that fat hangs over the top of them. I was motivated! Going to my closet I pulled out all my jeans which propelled me into action. What really hurt though was getting rid of my newly acquired white jeans with a silver pattern running up the sides of the legs. They were a size 2 which was psychologically thrilling to me who used to be a size 14. That's when Dr. Lebensohn said "Enough!

You must lose weight. You are pre-diabetic, have heart arrythmia, and high blood pressure according to your medical report."

I joined Weight Watchers after this wake-up call. I lost twenty pounds in the first year and have lost another twenty pounds since then, which I have kept off. Now everything seems normal. What a thrill! But the white jeans had to go. Besides they weren't comfortable, and I always had to pull them up. After ridding my closet and myself of ten pairs of jeans I was satisfied with the remaining jeans. They were 'mommy' jeans, but they were comfortable and flattering. I am sick and tired of tight, skinny jeans and have gravitated towards straight-legged jeans and am wondering if bell-bottoms will ever come back into vogue.

After the closet purge I set down and listened to music and gazed at my new wall hanging from the Food Bank Thrift Store. It is silver metal with orange leaves around the sides and bottom, and it says, "Live Simply and Remain Grateful." That is my new mantra. Living simply is fun, less confusing and not so destructive to our planet. I can't say enough about 'Remain Grateful.' For those of us on Planet Earth in 2021 it is awful to contemplate the devastation of our resources and environment which has been brought about by our inordinately driven desire for material items and throw-away items. Not to mention that there seem to be more people than we can presently sustain. I believe Father God and Mother Earth are possibly ending our stay on this planet.

Visualization

And then there is visualization: a great habit and one to be pursued relentlessly. What do I see or more to the point … in the past what did I see? I saw someone short and fat. I have never been beautiful. I am short which is the bane of my existence, but now that I am sure of God's love, I can even accept that. My body has been good to me and now I am returning the favor.

Today is Labor Day, September 6, 2021, and I am going to celebrate by going to the gym, do what Nick taught me and then go to volunteer at Hope Heals, an activity that makes my soul happy. I finally understand something I saw in Haiti while on a mission trip in January of 2010 when the devastating earthquake occurred. While walking through the town of Terre Haute, after working hard all day, we saw a young boy who was stark naked. My initial reaction or thought was that he was mentally ill. But after reflection it occurred to me that maybe his parents couldn't afford clothing for him. Then it occurred to me that perhaps he had no parents. I also observed that parents walked for miles to get their sick children to the clinic for medical help, something we mostly take for granted. I noticed how gracious these poor, afflicted people were.

Which brings me back to muffin tops ... so unflattering. After getting rid of my low-rise jeans (which only the young can pull off and it's iffy for them) from now on it's only mid-rise or above! It is sad to see how slovenly many people are ... young, middle-aged and old. I am especially saddened by the slovenly old who after many years of living and observing should have developed a sense of beauty and love of self. What is apparent is a lack of love of beauty and a love of self. Also lack of self-respect and anxiety, partially due to the loneliness and restrictions brought about the current covid pandemic. This could be an ongoing problem which we will need to learn to cope with. What has been hugely important to me is getting outside and walking. Therefore, I only have a tiny roll of excess skin around my mid-section.

Visualization: being able to see in the present where you are now, not living in the past and not foreseeing the future. Now is all we have. It can disappear and we will be no more. Gone for good from this planet and where we go depends a lot on what we believe. I visualize me being transported on a cloud with my musical instruments from cosmos to cosmos spreading the Gospel through music along with my musician friends ... like the Beatles.

Tights

It is apparent that almost everyone wears tights, including me. The main difference is I wear a tunic top which covers my rear end, or a dress or skirt. Line is important ... an unbroken line ... shades of the art department of William and Mary and Randy Michener of Manassas NOVA. A smooth line is comforting to the psyche and satisfies the longing for beauty. It goes along with what the designer said while fitting my first uniform, "Miss Goin, tight clothes are not quite nice."

Those words will resound in my mind forever. People today laugh when I tell them what he said but he seemed to have observed a profound truth. An unbroken, smooth line is soothing to the eye. It is beautiful and expressive. Rolls of fat are gross and expressive, just not in a flattering way. When I walked away from him in my newly fitted uniform, I felt attractive and was comfortable (able to move with ease) and was able to do both in a fashionable and stylish manner.

I have never forgotten these mind/life altering words. They have been the guiding light to my style sense. It gives me peace of mind to know my clothes slink over my body affording me ease of movement.

To this day my clothes must fall effortlessly from either my shoulders (if a dress) or from my waist (if a skirt or pants.)

As for tights they are mostly for exercise or modesty, especially if an article of clothing is too short. It all goes back to Twiggy who was extremely tall and thin and always looked good. She was my idea of the ideal fashionista and important to my way of thinking about how one should present themselves. I love tights but they need to feel slithery … and should come to either the calves or ankles to add an element of modesty which in today's culture is sorely needed.

They are fun to wear with large statement-shirts which to me are the ultimate source of fun in fashion. Many people have a great sense of fun and put it onto their t-shirts for men, women and children … short or tall, young or old, fat or thin. They are fun to wear and start many a conversation as modern Americans and others all notice them. I especially love my Snoopy (the ultimate dog) adorned apparel.

The Little Black Dress

What did Coco know? She knew about style! She knew that to be young at heart meant one had style, another word for 'love of beauty'. One can get old but remain young at heart and in spirit. I am biologically almost eighty (very old and as my brother says, "we are terminally tired." In my heart I am probably eight-ten years old ... The teen years seemed dreary except when indulging in adventures. The social scene was pure drudgery and worrying about my parents, especially my father, ruined nearly everything. To ease the pain there were clothes and books, both of which have fascinated me to this day.

Fortunately, I wasn't born in the ante-bellum South. The women's clothes were hideous in the extreme and excessively uncomfortable. Corsets were undoubtedly the most horrid form of clothing ever invented for women, rivaled only by foot-binding in China. They were intentionally meant to cripple women as was foot-binding. This hatred of women seems to be widespread and everlasting and is a hatred beyond my ability to comprehend. My grandmother wore a corset her entire life and compromised the strength of her back. To the end she even wore one to sleep in. Was this because of loss of strength or perceived vanity? This hatred probably could extend to girdles and stilettoes and pointy toe shoes which deform women's feet and backs.

The "little black dress" was made famous by Coco Chanel. I don't remember my first one, but it was probably when I went to work and had money which was promptly spent on clothes. When packing for a trip I usually took a black dress, a pair of jeans, a blazer or denim jacket, a white shirt, a bathing suit, walking shoes and dress shoes and a long t-shirt to sleep in.

This might seem boring, but I was happy and comfortable and looked good which appealed to my sense of good style and modernity. At that time of my life Nordstrom's came into being and I was forever after thrilled. Nordstoms was like a piece of Heaven come to Earth. Vive Nordstrom's!

The nice thing about a basic black dress is that it appeals to all fashion types and can be worn for almost any occasion, excepting formal affairs. It is slimming and becoming to most people and can be worn with about anything in the way of adornment. No one can forget Audrey Hepburn in her black dress in the great movie, "Breakfast at Tiffany's." She was sleek and gorgeous ... to be admired.

If you want to go to a formal affair nothing is more eye-catching than a slinky black formal gown. WOW!

Jeans!

Jeans are my favorite type of pants. I lost all interest in slacks and Bermuda shorts. It's denim all the way. Today jeans make up my outfit for most days of the week, usually worn with a t-shirt, and in cold weather, a jacket or blazer. Blouses are as unimportant to me as are slacks. Today I bought a pair of jeans at Marshall's which are so cool and make my legs look long and lean. They are so tight however that it's impossible to breathe so I will return them and continue the search. Lauren Conrad (one of my current style gurus) believes in buying multiples which I will consider in the future. That is hard for me as I tend to buy in consignment shops. There are several reasons for that:

1 ... it is cheaper and I no longer am interested in spending a lot of money on myself ..."live simply so that others may simply live" ...

2 ... it is environmentally a better deal all around ... for the water, for the earth, for the landfills

3 ... I don't drive much anymore, and malls and boutiques for the most part are unavailable.

Today I bought a neat jacket and would have bought another it, but it was too small. Many men and women are overweight and tend to buy clothes too small for them. This is especially true of jeans. The sizing has been changed so that psychologically people think they are wearing a smaller size. I can wear anything from an XS-XL, from a 2 to a 14. It is easier to shop if one's weight is at an acceptable level, basically achieved by not eating so much. Companies tend to mark sizes smaller than they should so that people will feel good about themselves and buy the smaller size. One should ignore the label and wear what looks good and is comfortable.

T-shirts are great with jeans. My favorites usually have a picture or a phrase on the front. My favorites feature Snoopy, Woodstock and NASA. I also like long shirts or ones cut off to the waist, hitting at the top of the hipbone.

With jeans I prefer a straight leg or boot cut. The in-style seems to be super- skinny which I am tired of. Legs that have flair and are fun and easy to wear are great. Bell bottoms were the ultimate but are out of vogue. But I am too short to wear them. And please: not super-low rise, unless you want to show muffin tops.

The Little Black Jacket

I am reading Lauren Conrad's "Style" and love it, especially the part about fashion and style. Her insight is great for one so young at the time she wrote it. She lists some items needed for good looks and warmth. One of these treasures is the "little black jacket."

I have several black leather jackets but until lately not a cloth one. It seems necessary, so I went 'a-hunting.' I found the perfect one at the Salvation Army and bought it, but when I got it home I decided it was too large which looks almost as bad as too small. It was too large, the sleeves were too long and I didn't think it worth altering. I took it to Hope Heals.

We hung it up and went about our job of sorting and hanging clothes when a little, old black lady came in. Lindsey told her we were closed for shopping, but the little lady was concerned about being around a lot of people as she was a candidate for covid. She was undergoing chemo and hadn't received her booster shot. Lindsey, being the great lady she is, told the little lady to go right ahead and not to mind us scurrying around. The little lady thanked her, grabbed a bag, signed in and started hunting.

I watched her and noticed how artfully she looked at everything and how careful she was to only pick items that suited her, and guess what! She found my black jacket, was thrilled that it fit and looked good on her. She carefully put it in her bag. Both she and I felt like a million bucks. God works in a mysterious fashion.

After carefully shopping for about an hour she thanked us, took her bag and departed. She was fun! She was having fun! I was having fun! Fun to me is one of the great blessings God has granted us.

I still needed a black jacket. My arms look better when covered and I get cold easily. A light-weight jacket is the answer, especially a black one. I went to Thrift Bank and as I found a beautiful Dana Buchman eyelet jacket which fit perfectly. Sheila and I thought it was perfect and would look great with my jeans and dresses. I know how the little, old, black lady felt when she discovered her perfect jacket.

Dr. Lebensohn understood human beings and the love of looking good that is prevalent in people of a sound mind. Looking good is fun and the thrill of the hunt is a part of the thrill. Sort of like a hunter finding a deer or moose which he shoots to provide food for his family. Hunting is a fun pursuit and a passion.

The Hunt

As Dr. Lebensohn advocated: "Hunt!" You don't need to buy unless something strikes you as necessary. That's what I do as the title of this book encourages. Hunting is the ultimate in fun for me and something I do every day I am mobile. It's also how I get out and associate with people which he said was a necessity. My hunt right now is for the perfect black jacket for the fall and winter. As I told you in the last chapter, this hunt was true for the little old black lady at Hope Heals. She was discriminating and in hope of looking stylish. She browsed with the utmost discretion, finding items perfect for her personality and style. The jacket was one of these items.

Now I need to find a black jacket for me. This is more difficult for me now as I have developed my eye and am more discriminating. There are two main reasons for this:

1 ... covid concerns me. Although my paranoia is in remission, I am aware that Russell and I are very old and vulnerable. Therefore, if there are many people in an area, I get out which limits my shopping

2 … I only drive around town or on occasion to Culpeper or Haymarket (about 30 minutes.) Yesterday I achieved the impossible and fulfilled two objectives: a … Shop Therapy and getting around people.

b … Julia Cameron says in "The Artist's Way" that once a week one should take 'an artist's date.' I took mine while attending a yard sale. It was fun and enjoyable to talk with the people at the sales. I went to Full Circle to look for things for Hope Heals and to find a black jacket for me.

I found a great pair of dark grey jeans and a black, silky, flowing top for 53 cents and a pair of black walking shoes which had never been worn for $2.00. I found an embellished denim jacket for $8 at Good Will. However, still no black jacket so I headed for Déjà vu where I found it! The ultimate black jacket with silver sparkles on the shoulders. It was too small. Oh, WOE! Sandra said it was too small and I trust her taste. She understands clothes, her customers and what suits them.

The immortal words of the designer of my first uniform formed my mind forever as he gazed deeply into my eyes and told me not to wear too tight, too small clothes. The 'hunt' continues and as the doctors have noticed I never give up. I will find it! I must! I trust!

He Sees the Beauty in Me

My heart belongs to Jesus, that's why my soul is free!

He sees the beauty in me!

Why, you may ask, is it important that my heart and soul belong to Jesus? Aside from the fact that His love for us, including me, 'saved' me. He set me free from worrying, being negative and most important, He showed me the relevance and importance of beauty, in myself and all surrounding me. Yes, there is ugliness, hatred, greed and the manipulation of others in this world but they no longer control my life and mind. I see the beauty of nature, of other species, of other people. This beauty carries over to how I present myself to the world … knowing that at any moment my life on Earth may be ended and I will be present in Heaven where I will see Him. As John 7:1 NKJV says: "Judge not that you be not judged", yet it is still important to present oneself as the most beautiful knowing that He loves beauty, and clothing and jewelry and our bodies are ways of showing this beauty.

To me it seems that when you don't care how you present yourself you are spitting in the face of the Creator. As for the beauty of nature take a walk and see for yourself. Look at the trees, listen to the birds and crickets, admire the markings of a garter snake if you are so fortunate as to see one.

It used to be that there were millions of bees, butterflies, grasshoppers, snakes, etc. but now it seems most of them have been exterminated. Are we really satisfied to be destroying our planet and its diversity of life and species which will ultimately end life on this planet? Dr. Wang transformed me when he explained to me that I was created by God as He thought beautiful that day. He loves me as a child of His. I was astounded. He also created the great diversity of life forms and species which he loves.

I started going to church and one morning Isabelle Jones, the organist, played "Great is Thy Faithfulness" which stirred my soul to be of service. It was the most beautiful music I had ever heard and to this day I love it more than any other song, even "Rock of Ages." Beauty! Beauty! Beauty! It's all around me and you, and the love of it is instilled deep into my being. It is the source of creativity, a gift from God to us and we hopefully will use this creativity to make a gift for Him and others.

Judge Not

"Judge not that you be not judged." Matthew 7:1(NKJV)

Dr. Lebensohn and Oscar Wilde said that you are judged and judged quickly by your appearance in a matter of seconds and that judgement is difficult to change. Almost all of us do it and we find it hard to change that initial judgement. But the Bible is explicit … don't judge so as not to be judged. Dr. Wang changed my life and made me happy. Dr. Lebensohn told me that in his experience people of sincere faith, especially followers of Christ, were the most likely to recover from brain dis-ease, perhaps because they had a 'rock' on which to stand … a foundation.

But I do judge. If people don't care enough to want to be and look their best (which doesn't mean expensive) then they don't care about themselves or others. The human psyche is complex and difficult to understand. However, looking good is a driving force (back to cave people) for most people of a sound mind. (2 Timothy 1:7 NKJV)). "God has not given us a spirit of fear, but a spirit of power and of love and of a sound mind."

Because I dress my best and strive to look attractive, all sorts of people start interesting conversations with me, including telling me how nice I look which brings a smile to my face and a "thank you" to my heart. I then tell others how nice they look which starts many a conversation and a smile to their face. There is so much uncertainty and fear in the world that such a little thing as a sincere compliment brings a moment of ease and happiness.

One type of clothing popular today which tells oodles about a person's heart and mind is the t-shirt with a slogan or picture on it. I love them. My favorites are:

1 ... style is free

2 ... life is too short to wear boring clothes

3 ... anything with Snoopy and Woodstock

People who think often pride themselves on wearing a shirt which celebrates what they believe. I love to read them as much as I love to read bumper stickers. Businesses use t-shirts as a uniform today much as I wore a uniform when I went to work. Uniforms give a 'uniform' appearance as well as a source of advertisement. I love to read t-shirts and am aware of how clever or effective they are. Can't get away from judging!

Style Mentor

I found a wonderful old cartoon from Parade Magazine, 1985, in which a gangster is lying on the couch, scowling, as his psychiatrist says, "Get out and meet people, make new accomplices." It makes me smile to look at it, and it reminds me of my relationships with my doctors and counselors telling me to meet new people, especially the part about new accomplices.

I lost Rosemary many years ago but have found a new mentor. Her name is Sandra and she is the proprietress of a great consignment shop in town, Déjà vu. She is from Germany and the mother of three ... the possessor of a grand eye for style (my art professor, Randy, also has this great eye.) She has a wonderful ability to help her clients develop their own personal style, to look their best and to seemingly do it effortlessly. She helps them look their best relatively inexpensively and as a recycler she and they both help the planet.

She has great charm, beauty and gorgeous black hair which sometimes is blue, purple, etc. It is sometimes longer, sometimes shorter. Like me, she is a crow ... likes anything that sparkles and glitters. She likes t-shirts with a picture or slogan, and she likes distressed jeans. She hires young ladies (teenagers) to help in her store. She encourages them to venture into the world traveling lightly and following adventure.

Her kids are great, following MaMa's footsteps. They each have a unique way of presenting themselves. I told Sandra about Russell's comment about distressed clothes one afternoon while we were chit-chatting. He said that when men find their jeans too disgustingly ugly to wear, they throw them into the trash and women retrieve them and wear them with love and devotion. He said that "it is sometimes embarrassing to be seen with you!" And in relation to the cartoon, he observed that "it is disturbing to know your sister was a moll." Now I am such a priss, but even back then God loved me which I know because he got me such wonderful doctors who were forward thinking. They healed a sick mind and a wounded, lost spirit.

From them I learned the importance of being kind to one's fellow beings. Some studies show that kind people are happier and live longer if I understand them correctly.

Recovery From a State of Disarray

"Disarray, Dr. Lebensohn? You say I am in disarray! What should I do?" Me and my mind were in a quandary, so as a woman of 'steely determination' I set out to discover the 'real' me—whatever that should be—and my soul guides were Twiggy and Rosemary. Later in the 90's it would be the sales ladies in the French, Belgium, English and German designer shops. The sales ladies were probably the most important because they taught me about recycling and the value of consignment shops. My mother and grandmother were horrified at the mere thought of wearing 'used' clothing, something 'not new' but it seemed foolish to me to spend a fortune which I didn't have for clothes when there were not only consignment shops but shops like Zara, H and M, and Top Shop.

My great doctor also stressed the importance of not wearing stilettoes or spike heels and pointy toed shoes if I wanted to preserve the integrity and health of my back and feet. Except for going to and from the airplane I never again wore shoes of that type. I can still walk up to five miles a day and have relatively good posture which makes me look taller, more like Twiggy … a dream for me impossible to achieve.

Then something happened to the world which is not easy to comprehend. Was it 9/11? Impossible to say for certain but it seemed that the airlines and our country in general began a decline into being a police state, and a false sense of security and safety started to take the place of democracy. The food industry continued selling and advertising quick and highly processed food. Now almost 75% of the world's human population is overweight or obese ... a disturbing trend that seems to have contributed to the general state of 'slobbism.' I fell into the trap until Dr. Lebensohn told me to lose the excess pounds as I was pre-diabetic, had high blood pressure and a disturbed heart.

After joining Weight Watchers, I lost nearly twenty pounds, gave up being a vegan and lost another seventeen pounds, and regained my health. Under Dr. Lebensohn's guidance I once again became stylish. Here is a quote from the November/December 1998 Weight Watchers magazine from Ms. Laura Fraser who hid from the world in drab clothes until the owner of a chic boutique in San Francisco took over her approach to appearance and style. Here is a quote which is important for us all: "If my Marijha's makeover taught me anything, it's that fabulous has nothing to do with my size and everything to do with showing the world who I really am."

Thank you Marijha, Rosemary, Sandra and salesladies the world over. May you "live long and prosper."

A Big Heart

My quote from yesterday was brought to life today at Marshalls ... fabulous has nothing to do with size and everything to do with showing the world who I really am."

I was standing in line behind a black lady who was excessively fat, but that's not what I noticed. What did I notice? Her weight was making her uncomfortable, but she was beautiful despite her weight and discomfort. She was wearing a pair of slightly distressed midnight blue jeans with perfectly, strategically placed rhinestone twinkles. Her t-shirt was white cotton and slightly long with long sleeves pushed back to the elbows showing silver bangle bracelets and beautifully manicured nails. The front of the t-shirt had in large letters the word "LOVE" emblazoned with rhinestones to match the jeans. She had a beautifully shaped head adorned with a short, black, 1-inch- long Afro and beautiful brown eyes ... a lovely, lovely woman of an indeterminant age. It was hard to determine her age, but she obviously had a gentle and loving spirit.

After I left Marshalls I went up town to the Festival. As I walked down the street, I noticed most of the people ... men, women, children ... were slobs. What made the difference? Obviously the people on the street didn't care about themselves and others while the lady at Marshalls did care. I will never forget her and her beautiful heart and spirit. I pray I present myself as well.

That was my lesson about a big heart. She was undoubtedly the loveliest lady I have ever seen ... sort of like the big Hawaiian ladies I saw while living in Hawaii in their colorful muumuus, which I hate but which suited them to perfection. They were huge and decked out in wildly colored and patterned muumuus. They also appeared beautiful and happy to the world around them. Like the lady at Marshalls, I will never forget them ... ladies of the sun and sea.

All of them were people of great hearts. Not only did they fulfill Dr. Lebensohn's theory that one is judged in seconds and will often not be able to change the impression they first made. All I know is that it would make me glad to cause others to have that impression of me ... the impression Miss Big Heart made on me. God Bless Her!

More Fun, Less Stuff

This philosophy sums up my latest and greatest approach to living. Fun has always been important to me which is why the Way of Christ means so much to the way I live and go about my business. Jesus enjoyed life and the people. He loved beauty. According to the Bible when he was crucified the soldiers gambled for possession of his robe. They considered it either beautiful or useful, not to be destroyed. Lloyd C. Douglas even wrote his book "The Robe" about it.

Which reminds me: I must go to Hope Heals this morning and see if the beautiful Italian jacket is still there. It is too small for me but is gorgeous and I want to look at it again. Its simple beauty is a source of joy to me.

Live Simply! I talked to Dr. Goldstein yesterday. He is 75 and we both feel our age. He was concerned I might be lonely if Russell should die before me. I am not lonely. Sometimes I am disgruntled by my relationships, so I change them to something more satisfying. That generally means the more satisfying friend likes to look at stuff. As we are getting older and seeing all the 'stuff' out there, it is becoming less important to buy and own it as there is not enough room for it.

I got a card from Nature Conservancy which sums up my current approach to 'stuff':

1 … showcase simple beauty using items from Nature to bring color and beauty into your home

2 … eat more veggies and fruit. I did not say no animal products, just more plant food.

3 … purchase wisely and recycle

4 … reduce plastic waste. This idea has revolutionized the way I think and shop.

5 … repurpose and reuse. Things don't have to be new to be useful and hopefully they won't end up in the landfill.

6 … shop locally, both farmers and regular merchants. This also reduces the use of fossil fuels. Local markets are fun and get you out and around others.

All these ideas lead to "More Fun, Less Stuff" which leads to having more fun. The 'hunt' is exciting and interesting. It leads to better style because one thinks more about what one is doing and buying. It helps to develop a better eye for quality, both of materials and design.

As for the 'stuff' in my room … it is so soothing to my mind-body. Especially my rocking chair which is from around 1850 and still beautiful. It is fun to rock away the 'blues' if I get them.

How to Help Nature

God and Mother Nature will undoubtedly have the last word, and it is up to us to do our part to restore the health of our planet. I was in Kohls looking at the young girl's department where I saw a neat yellow, hooded shirt which said, "Save the bees." I nearly cried. This summer I saw only 3 bees including the carpenter bees which usually are all over the place. While I was walking this evening, I saw my third lightning bug. I have only seen one grasshopper in Russell's yard since 2006. This is so sad, an indication of the destruction that has going on, largely due to pesticides, herbicides and other toxic poisons … thank you Montsanto and your Round Up.

In our decorating we can showcase Nature's beauty. I have 3 dried arrangements which have been made from plants gathered on my walks. One of them is a brown Chinese cat ceramic pillow which has cattails sticking out of a hole at the tail of the cat. It is at least 30 years old. I haven't seen a cattail in years. Another arrangement is a black metal cat filled with items of nature picked up on my walks, red plastic berries and a Christmas decoration which was too pretty to throw away. The third arrangement is 'weeds' stuck into a gorgeous green vase I picked up at the Thrift Bank. Those proceeds go to help those who are food deprived.

We should eat more plant food. We need animal products, in my opinion, but we need less to lower our carbon footprint.

We should purchase wisely and recycle, keeping in mind that often there is excessive packaging which is unnecessary. We should reduce plastic waste as so much of it goes into the ocean, killing our ocean life. I suggest to store- managers that they accommodate people who use reusable cups and glasses. They might need to charge a little more, but it is worth it. We should repurpose and reuse, like the blender and food processor I bought used and have been using for several years …"One man's junk is another man's treasure."

As much as possible shop locally. I buy as much food as I can from Alvin Henry who has a great little market down the street. His products are reasonably local, seasonal and reasonably priced.

Have fun looking and only buy when something is wonderful. I get rid of something when I get something new, and most of my stuff I love. One doesn't need to buy just to be buying.

Live Simply, Remain Grateful

It's the only rewarding way to live, bringing satisfaction on a deep level. It helps those around you which is what God commands: Jesus said to him, "You shall love the Lord your God with all your heart, with all your soul and with all your mind. This is the first and great commandment. And the second is like unto it: You shall love your neighbor as yourself ..." (Matthew 22: 37-39 NKJV). I have found that giving is of the utmost value—of resources, time and money ... to love others. It is of great importance to love our planet and all its inhabitants ... flowers, trees, rivers, mountains, animals, birds, fish and insects. Everything was created by God, and each has a reason for being given to them by Him.

Dr. Wang gave me hope when there was none, and he gave me the knowledge that there was a purpose for my life, and that God created and loved me. Adventure was fine, and greatly to be desired and admired, but has brought me nowhere the satisfaction I have derived from church, volunteering at the Book Cellar and Hope Heals...and looking one's best.

Is this sheer vanity? I think it's important because I believe our body is the temple of the Holy Spirt and as such deserves all the consideration we can give it. It is pure fun, bringing pleasure throughout one's lifetime. It gives the ability to move about freely, using our senses freely. To have these abilities is reason to be thankful and to be grateful every day of our lives, including the desire to share this joy with others and to help those less fortunate.

So many people today do not care about themselves or others or the world we inhabit. It seems we are gleefully destroying our environment and its inhabitants. Why is a puzzle to me as it is a fact that we have the brains and intellect to take care of what we have been given, and to share. LIVE SIMPLY! DO NOT WASTE RESOURCES!

When I wear something I ask myself as I take it off: "Do I love it enough to wear it again?" If not, I donate it to Full Circle, Hope Heals, Deja Vu, Treasure Box, Salvation Army, Good Will, Thrift Bank, etc. I get something from them in return. It is fun to 'hunt' ... to participate in Shop Therapy. I enjoy Dr. Lebensohn's advice to look and enjoy beauty, not always to buy and to send this 'stuff' to others to enjoy, even to people in other countries. The "hunt" is popular around the world and throughout the history of existence.

"Remember to Look Up at the Stars

So said Stephen Hawking. What a beautiful thought! I looked at my painting of the stars and a telescope, put on my black leather jacket and stepped out onto the deck. I saw the moon, not quite full, but bright and lighting up the early morning sky. It was cold as fall has started. My jacket is smart and warm. I got it at Hope Heals. It was my gift to myself for working all morning. It fits to perfection. Recycling clothes is great fun for me and enables me to give to others who are in need.

Some days when I go to Hope Heals with Deb to look, I notice the same people at the Thrift Bank Food Store the next day hoping to get food. Sobering! My heart bleeds for them. Is it our system, is it lack of education? What causes this mess that is going on all over the world, even in the USA which is the richest country in the history of the world? In my more negative moments, it seems that perhaps there are more people than the planet can support.

Watching the little black lady shop last week was so encouraging for me. She was meticulous about how she looked and shopped artfully, taking only what she needed and what looked good on her. She knew her style. Unlike the young woman who was shopping with her mother. She was at least a size 14 or 16 but couldn't accept the fact and kept taking 2's and 4's. Her mother tried to get her to take clothes that would fit her but obviously she couldn't accept the fact she was so big. It saddened me because she rejected a gorgeous dress that would have looked elegant on her because it was 'too big.'

This kind of thinking has become so prevalent that many companies put smaller labels on their clothes because it makes people feel better about how they look … sort of like the current acceptable weight ranges. They are around 10 pounds heavier than when I was young.

Back then, in the airlines, we were so thin but were required to wear a girdle. Today when they are needed it is almost impossible to find one. I haven't seen one in years. 'Too tight' is considered sexy.

I have discovered that when someone looks nice, I say something to them, and people open start conversations with me to tell me when they think I look nice. Sincere compliments bring a smile to the face and a laugh to the heart.

The Squirrel with an Inch Long Tail

Russell and I enjoy sitting on the deck in the late afternoon, watching the birds, squirrels and rabbits eat and frolic and bathe in the bird bath. When the dozens and dozens of blackbirds took over, Russell stopped feeding the birds. All the critters seemed to be mad at Russell, and for a month or so we set on the deck and saw no one. Finally, they started coming back and one of the critters was a squirrel with only about an inch long tail. Horrors! Squirrels seem to be rats with long, bushy tails with which they must communicate and use for balance. This unfortunate squirrel had no tail to speak of. Was he born that way or did an animal or car break it off? We'll never know, but for sure he looks wrong.

I used to watch Nick Vuicicik on Christian TV. He was born with only a head and torso ... no arms or legs. His parents obviously had the money to raise him and help him develop a wonderful personality and spirit of helpfulness. He was fun to listen to and he traveled all over the world speaking to audiences of possibly millions of people, telling them about how God used him to help others. I loved listening to him but haven't seen him in a long while. Has he died? I will have to check into that.

Like the squirrel (despite his handicap) he developed friends and a playful spirit. Our squirrel plays with his buddies, climbs up trees (right side up and upside down), drinks at the bird bath, eats the corn and generally frolics and seems to have a good time with his fellow squirrels, birds and rabbits. Like Nick and many other souls, he has learned to be happy despite his disadvantage. Russell and I have stopped feeling sorry for him and observe his antics with glee. Like the squirrel with the blond tail, he has become instantly recognizable to us. The other squirrels look alike and are not recognizable although they too are unique. But this animal stands apart not only because of his disfigurement but because of his playful and friendly personality.

Like this squirrel so many of my fellow humans have overcome disadvantages to live in harmony with others and to alter others' initial impression of disfavor to become a source of joy and even beauty in their uniqueness.

My Being—Who I Am

Why is this important in a book about appearance? When you appear to others you are saying "this is my being." This is who I am?" If you look like a slob you are saying to those who see you who you are. Appearance is our way of showing our identity.

Today I wore my black sweatpants with Tim Burton's 'the nightmare before Christmas" characters running up the side of the leg, and a black t-shirt with a pink and green frog saying "fully rely on God." My minister even started a conversation about the frog and his words. He is concerned about the loss of parishioners due to covid and how it is affecting the future of the church. That is his way of asking for our prayers. He agreed with what Frog had to say.

Nothing particularly subtle about this outfit but it draws attention in a fun- loving way, making one accessible to others. Dr. Lebensohn said to talk to people, and I would discover three things:

1 … I like most people

2 … Most people have problems

3 ... Half of those have problems worse than mine.

There are evil people but stay away from them. They must take responsibility for their words, actions and the misery, hatred and fear they embody. Covid is not responsible for what they choose to be, but it has been instrumental in getting them to show their true colors ... nothing subtle about them. They obviously don't care about others and do not care about themselves, usually only money and power and the use of others. They don't care about family or friends. I remember when the polio vaccine first came out, we all eagerly got the shot or took the pill. There was no yammering about our 'rights' being ignored and the government inserting 'chips' under our skin to control us. As one who suffered from acute paranoia, I feel qualified to recognize paranoia when I see it. I also know how damaging it is to others and one's ability to function positively in society. Is that what you want for your identity? Is that "who I am?" It would seem the answer is 'yes.'

Love to be Me

That's a thought I heard. A thought! Could such a simple thing like a thought influence my presentation? Yes! It seems that is true and has lasting repercussions for me and my peers. When I was in college one day sitting at a window, observing the passing world (at the Wigwam, the campus coffee shop and hangout) a Bible verse popped into my head (Habbakuk 2:4 NKJV) ... "Behold the proud. His soul is not upright in him. But the just shall live by his faith." I didn't really understand these verses but have never forgotten them ... Now they make sense to me. They have always come to me to give me hope for the future and a reason to live even when things are darkest. How does this affect my presentation and my concept of the body as the 'temple of the Holy Spirit?'

It seems that as I age life is more fun and inspiring. My vision has always been to be graceful and lean. Being thin has always been important and it requires serious effort and diligence, especially to be neither to be too fat nor too thin. Anorexia for me is a serious hazard. Years of flying when you could be fired for being overweight led to poor self-image and dangerous eating habits, leading to anorexia nervosa. After quitting smoking, I became seriously overweight. Enter Weight Watchers. After many years I am slim, trim, healthy.

I believe God wants us to be healthy. Sometimes our life is complicated … often by stress, anxiety and depression. Nick Viucicik, despite being only a head and torso, became a world- famous evangelist. I believe he has written a book which I will check out at Open Book. I love books as much as I love clothes. That's the reason I volunteer at the Book Cellar and Hope Heals. As Edward Bulwer-Lytton said in the 1800's, "the pen is mightier than the sword."

If your mind is filled with encouraging thoughts (read Charles Schultz's "Peanuts.") then your face is happy, and a smile fills your heart. People feel encouraged when they look at you. Your expression is as important as your physical appearance. It took Dr. Wang to give me faith which appears in the verse above, "The just shall live by faith."

So, I shall plod along, day by day. Living for the moment means that what we do now, today, influences our future, perhaps making it meaningful and maybe even prosperous. But the main thing is to love life.

Clothe Thy Neighbor as Thyself

Before ending this book, I wish to address what I saw on a bumper sticker at the Methodist Church yesterday: "Clothe thy neighbor as thyself." That slogan on the car stopped me dead in my tracks as I was taking my morning amble around my neighborhood. I know the Bible says, "You shall not hate your brother in your heart. You shall surely rebuke your neighbor and not bear sin because of him. You shall not take vengeance, no bear any grudge against the children of your people, but you shall love your neighbor as yourself. I am the Lord." (Leviticus 19:17-18 NKJV) which seems to be an all-encompassing concept, but I had never considered my part in clothing others as part of showing my love for them.

I went home and went through my two small closets which were packed with clothing. Since clutter is disgusting to me, I rid myself not only of things which no longer fit or I was tired of, but those items I love which would enhance the life of someone less fortunate than me of whom there are plenty.

I got rid of all my distressed jeans which seem inappropriate and would be perfect for a junior or someone younger. I got rid of several gorgeous jackets because it is getting cold and warmth is important to having a tranquil mind/body. I got rid of dresses, t-shirts, etc. because I don't need them and possibly they will bring pleasure to someone else because I do have good taste. This good taste and good eye have been made possible thanks to the efforts of many ladies and gentlemen of taste I have encountered throughout my gallivanting around the world.

Dr. Lebensohn is dead now and probably Dr. Wang, and Dr. Goldstein is getting up there in age and will probably retire soon. I will still have Cindy and Autumn to keep me on the straight and narrow, plus whoever Dr. Goldstein will recommend. I have learned about life, love, adventure and kindness from them … also the love of reading, especially the KJN and NKJV versions of God's Word and Mikhail Bulgakov's "The Master and Margarita." The importance of faith, purpose and development of the mind/body have all played an important part in my living a long, productive and happy life for which I thank them.

And to end this book it seems vitally necessary to say what I have learned:

1 … treat your body and mind with respect and honor

2 … do not judge others if possible

3 … present yourself as best you can to cheer up the world you inhabit

4 … do not speak ill of others and try not to think ill of them

5 … SMILE!

Psalm 30: 10-13 NKJV

Hear, O Lord, and have mercy on me: Lord, be my helper!
You have turned for me my mourning into dancing;
You have put off my sackcloth and clothed me with gladness,
To the end that my glory may sing praise to You and not be silent.
O Lord my God, I will give thanks to You forever.

The End!

Printed in the United States
by Baker & Taylor Publisher Services